See how yoga fee

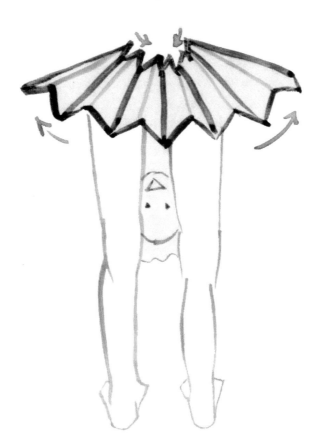

Visualisations to help the practice of yoga

by Su Sareen

I would like to take this opportunity to thank all those wonderful and
generous people who have helped me on my yoga journey so far.
I owe particular thanks to: Vanda Scaravelli, Daphne Pick, Lolly Stirk,
John Stirk, Sandra Sabatini, Rosie Mills, Carrie Tuke, Andrea Schaverien, Sue Aron,
Anne-Marie Zulkahari, Israela Butterworth, Sandra Jacobs and Elizabeth Herr.
A special thank you to Rick.

ISBN: 144145814X
EAN13: 9781441458148

VISUALISATIONS TO HELP
THE PRACTICE OF YOGA

The experience of practising yoga is an internal one.
It's about your relationship with your own body, developing an
awareness that goes way beyond the practice itself. So this book
concentrates on the inner experience and uses the fact that simply by
imagining things about your body, you can make them really happen.
This is true for all styles of yoga and for beginners right through
to advanced students and teachers.

This book is a practical guide.
The aim is to help you with useful visualisations that can
actually support you in the postures. It can be used by anyone who
practises yoga, alongside other books and classes to help
deepen understanding and enrich your practice.

Yoga should be an enjoyable experience.
I hope using this book will be enjoyable too.

CONTENTS

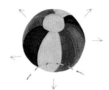
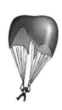

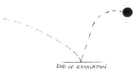

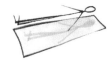

SECTION 2: SOME POSTURES

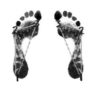

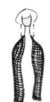
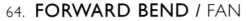
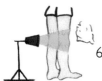

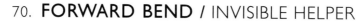 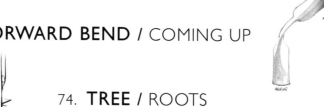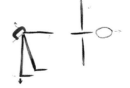
 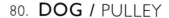
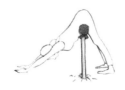

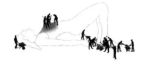
 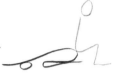
 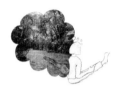
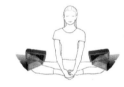 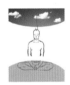

WHY DO YOGA?

The rewards are not only huge - but often unexpected.
Hatha yoga (the postures) looks like physical exercise
and its practice is certainly good for the body.
But that's just the beginning - once your mind and body start
working as one, you will experience real long-tem benefits:

You will have an altogether different relationship with your body
and, to a much greater extent, you'll be the one in charge.

You will grow old with a straighter spine and a degree of health and
sheer comfort in your body usually only enjoyed by the young.

You will develop your focus - an ability you'll find improves
your performance in many unexpected ways!

You will be better able to deal with the shocks that impact your
body without allowing trauma to create even more pain.

You will become more in charge of your whole self - mind and body -
through sheer awareness, feeling stronger and more alive.

ABOUT THIS BOOK

Why practice yoga? Rather than just master advanced or impressive positions, I would love to grow old with a straighter spine and the flexibility and comfort in my body that we all enjoyed as children. That's why this book covers mostly just the basic postures and concentrates on the simplest.

While everyone's yoga practice inevitably keeps developing, for me, some themes remain constant - like listening to and working with the body rather than forcing it; paying total attention to experiencing my yoga practice while being supported by the breath and gravity; simply witnessing what is and accepting it.

The book is split into two main sections:
Section One contains general principles, insights and ideas that are relevant to virtually all of the postures... things like the breath and gravity. Many observations here came originally from Scaravelli, but will be useful to practitioners from all yoga backgrounds.

Section Two contains posture visualisations.
You won't find all of the positions here and some are covered in more depth than others. For example, there is a lot on standing as it's the basic start point for many other postures.

This book assumes a basic knowledge of the postures and is best used alongside other books and classes.

SECTION 1: GENERAL PRINCIPLES

This section contains some big ideas - discoveries and insights that should be helpful throughout your whole practice.

When teaching, and when working on my own I weave these fundamental thoughts, insights and observations throughout.

Gathered together in this section you'll find:

- a bit about starting
- various ways of looking at the breath (not pranayama, breathing exercises are not covered in this book)
- a few observations about gravity
- why roots are so important when stretching
- a way of thinking about the spine
- a challenge... about managing your attention

At the very beginning of a practice, no matter
whether you're starting lying down, standing
or any other way, the moment your yoga
practice really begins is when you take
your whole attention fully inside
your body, letting go
of everything else.

It's total immersion
- just like diving
into deep
water.

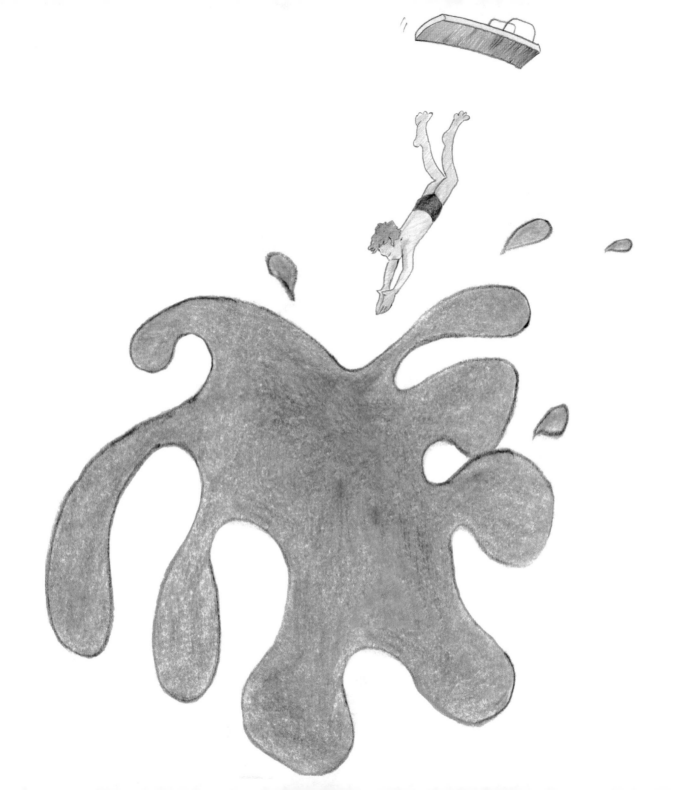

...and having jumped in, imagine that you have become the lake itself.

Settling in will have created disturbance - not just on the surface but throughout the body.
As you start your practice, watch dispassionately as the whole body comes to stillness,
starting at the surface and then gradually becoming quieter, deeper, deeper
and deeper still with every exhalation.

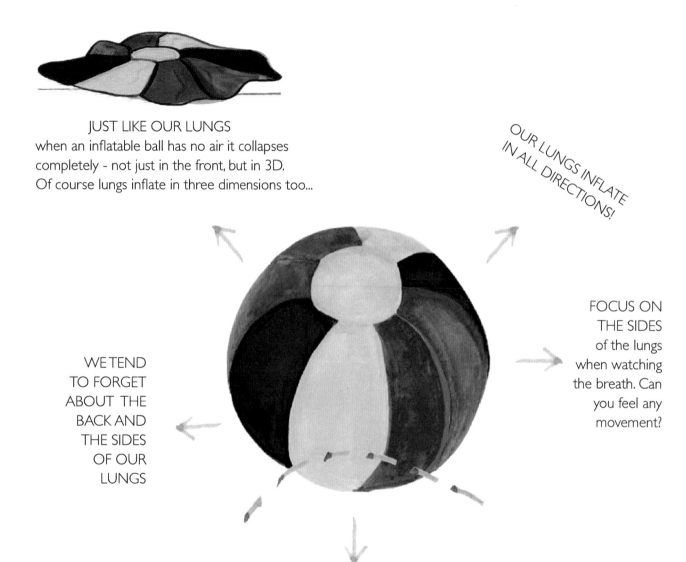

JUST LIKE OUR LUNGS
when an inflatable ball has no air it collapses
completely - not just in the front, but in 3D.
Of course lungs inflate in three dimensions too...

OUR LUNGS INFLATE IN ALL DIRECTIONS!

**FOCUS ON
THE SIDES**
of the lungs
when watching
the breath. Can
you feel any
movement?

**WE TEND
TO FORGET
ABOUT THE
BACK AND
THE SIDES
OF OUR
LUNGS**

THE BASE OF THE LUNGS
is probably the most important area to focus on while watching the breath.
It's the diaphragm. See if you can feel it moving as you breathe.

SIMPLY BY
IMAGINING
THINGS ABOUT
OUR BODY

WE CAN
MAKE THEM
REALLY
HAPPEN

EMPTY YOUR MIND
INTO YOUR EXHALATION

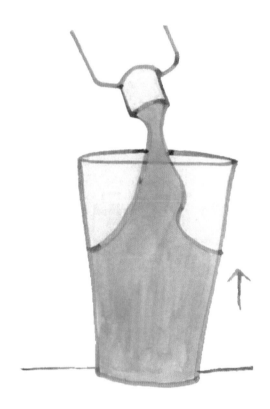

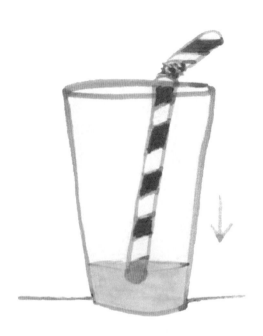

AS YOU BREATHE IN

picture your lungs receiving the air
into the base of the lungs first.
Watch them fill up just like a glass of water fills
- from the bottom up.
Don't allow the air to fill your lungs all the
way to the top. Even when practising breathing
exercises, leave the very tops of your lungs empty
and keep your breath comfortably within limits.

AS YOU BREATHE OUT

visualise the air leaving your lungs
from the top first; just like the level
of liquid in a glass drops from the
top downwards when it's being
sucked out by a straw.

Notice that the last part of the lung to
empty is the base (the diaphragm).

At the base of the lungs is the vitally important diaphragm - effectively the bottom wall of the lungs, it's a huge muscle that separates the chest cavity from the abdominal cavity. The diaphragm lies more or less at the very centre of our bodies and, as the muscle of respiration, moves hugely with the breath.

So it is a direct physical connection between the breath and the body.

In terms of shape and movement, think of the diaphragm like a parachute that becomes slightly deflated by the inhalation (pushed downwards) and is pulled upwards into the rib cage, inflating as it fills with the exhalation.

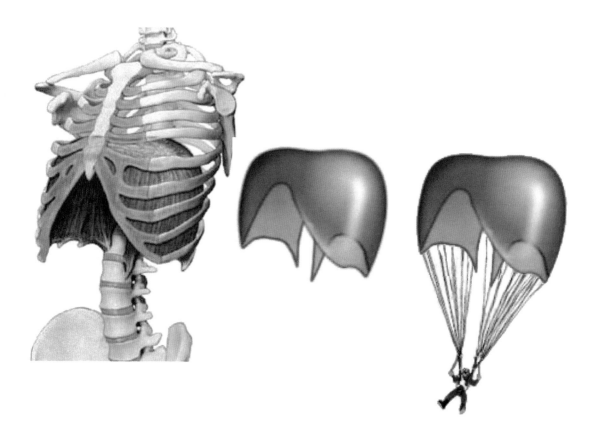

INHALATION

As the breath comes in, the diaphragm moves downwards and the air is pulled into the lungs, inflating them outwards in all directions.

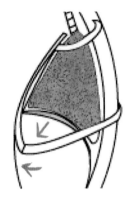
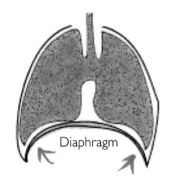

Diaphragm

EXHALATION

As the air leaves the lungs, the diaphragm moves upwards into the parachute shape. The lungs deflate as the air is pushed out.

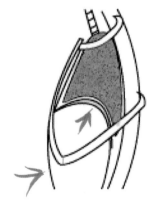
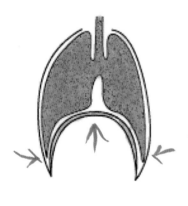

Importantly, the diaphragm is also connected to the deep abdominal muscles, which are connected to the front of the spine.

There's a rebound - a kind of ripple effect
that happens naturally at the end of an exhalation.
The problem is we can't DO it.
Instead, look for the precise moment which
marks the very end of an exhalation.
Be completely relaxed and attentive to your spine.

See if you can notice the snake-like micro-movements
that are your spine's response to your breath.

The strength of any rebound depends entirely on the strenth of the initial impact - the harder something is thrown, the stronger the bounce...

...so the more strongly you concentrate on noticing the exact moment at the very end of an exhalation, the more you'll feel the effect.

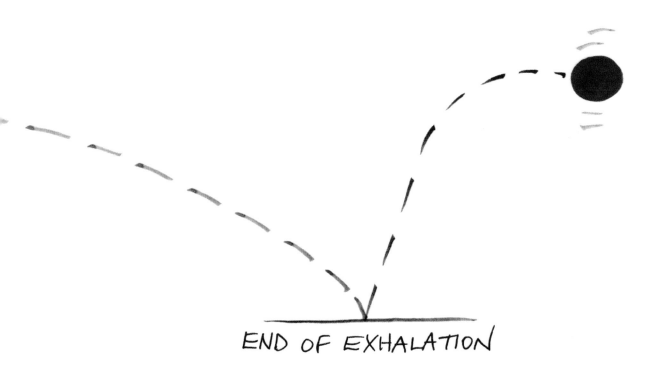

END OF EXHALATION

The idea is very simple - the breath spirals around the spine.
Work alternately with the inhalation and the exhalation, imagining the
breath spiralling up and around the spine as you breathe in and down
and around the spine as you breathe out.

Play around with your spirals to find what works best for you -
it may feel more natural if the spirals stay small and close to the spine.
At other times it may feel wonderful to sit within an energy that's
spiralling around your body.

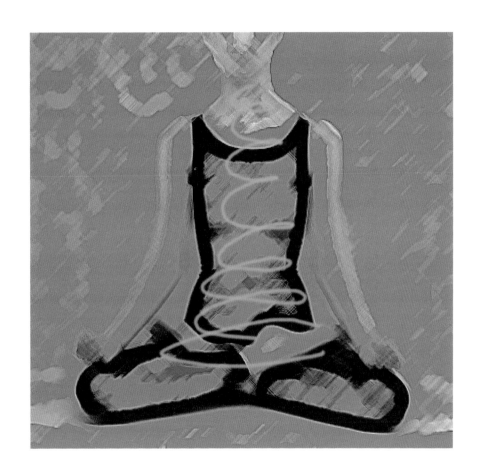

Shown sitting here, this breathing visualisation works just as well lying down and can even be effective in some standing postures.

This is impossible.
PROVE IT TO YOURSELF
for the teeniest moment try floating just 1mm above the ground.

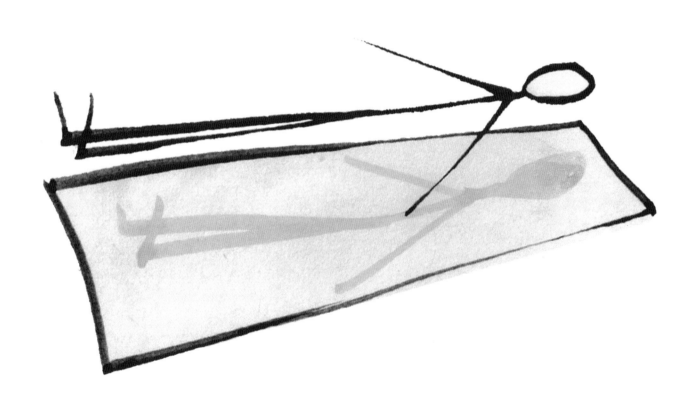

RESISTANCE IS USELESS!

Looking at it another way, we all
already know how powerful gravity is,
otherwise we'd jump off high buildings!

So rather than resisting, put all your effort
into going WITH gravity - embrace it.

Welcome gravity and it becomes a key
tool - one of the strongest and most useful.

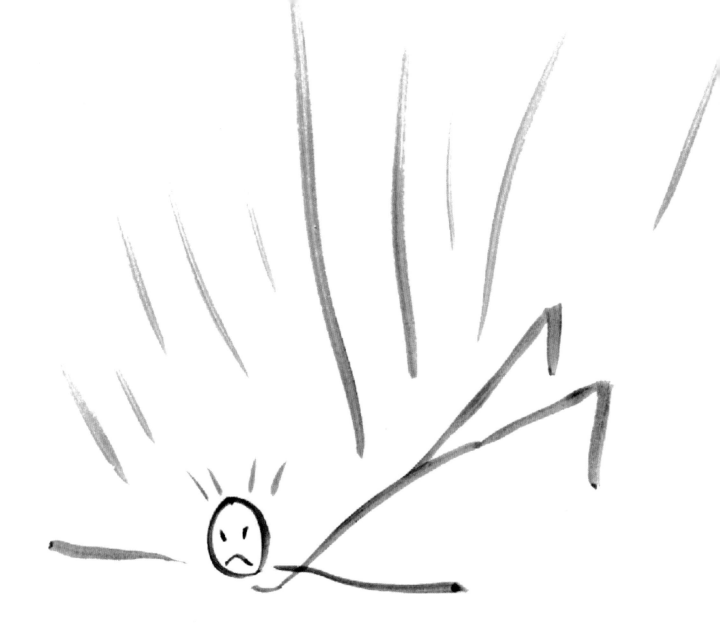

NEVER UNDERESTIMATE GRAVITY

We are so weedy and out-classed in the face of gravity, it's rather relaxing! As you lie resting on the floor, enjoy giving yourself up completely to the huge pull.

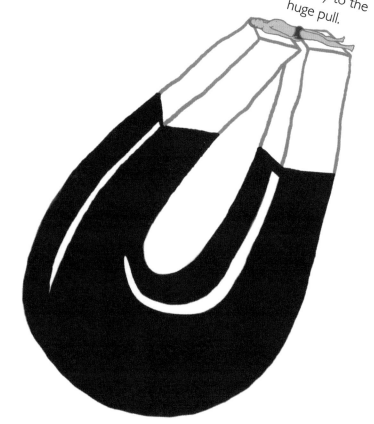

BECOME
THE
RHYTHM
OF
YOUR
BREATH

GIVE YOURSELF UP TO THE GROUND

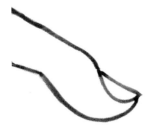

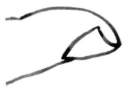

A CHALLENGE:

Using just one hand, try stretching a piece of elastic...

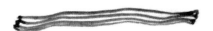

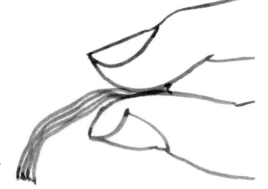

...hmmmm.

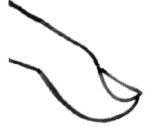

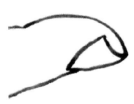

Try stretching the same piece of elastic
again, but now held in place by a pin...

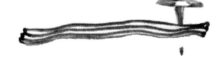

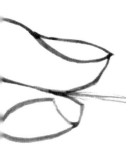

EASY!
But notice that even elastic will
not stretch without being held...

...and, within limits, the more
securely a piece of elastic is held,
the further it will stretch.

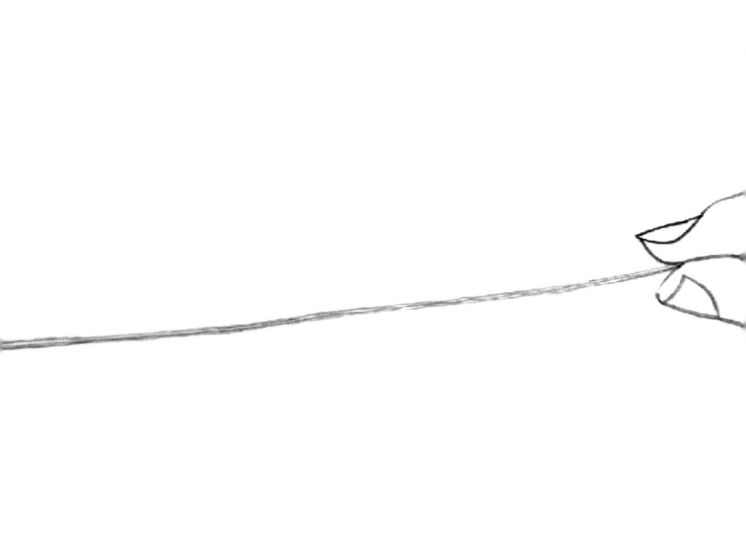

Your
spine is not
one long bone, it's
lots of little ones.
They have the potential
to move independently
and when they do,
the movement is snake-like,
rippling up and down the spine.
If you can soften the
deep muscles around
the spine and pay close
attention, you'll notice the
spine making lots of these
tiny 'micro-movements'
all without your
'doing
it'.

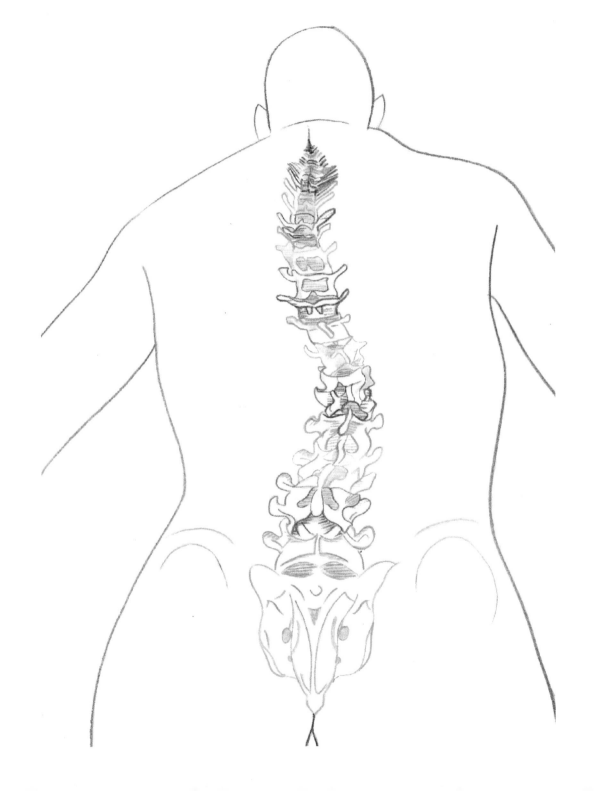

KEEPING OUR ATTENTION
ON WHAT WE ARE DOING
AS WE ARE DOING IT
IS THE MAIN
CHALLENGE IN YOGA

It may help to think of your attention as if it were a young and eager puppy;

our attention also seems to want to
run ahead of us - we can feel that we're
continually trying to keep up with it...

Call your attention to heel so that it follows what is happening
rather than trying to lead. Over time, you'll find you've trained
it into staying with you for longer and longer.

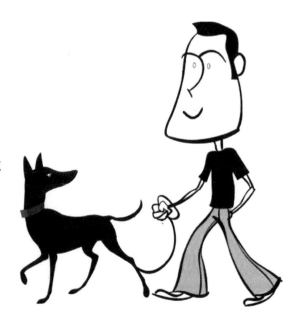

SECTION 2 / SOME POSTURES

This section shows visualisations as they might be used in the context of various common postures.
Many of the ideas expressed easily translate to other postures - for example, the idea of roots is invaluable in many standing and sitting postures as well as balances and inverted postures ...in fact, wherever your body meets the ground. The thing is just to play around with the ideas.

I teach and practice many postures not shown here.
But as my ultimate goal is to maintain a high degree of comfort and mobility in my body as I age, it's the quality of my attention rather than the level of difficulty of the postures that I strive to improve.

TADASANA

We really can open our feet.
This not only feels great, but gives a
bigger, firmer, more secure base.

Although it's our toes that move most obviously,
the opening comes from the centre of the foot -
it can feel like a flower opening.

Try playing with opening your feet and toes in
the bath when they're nice and warm.

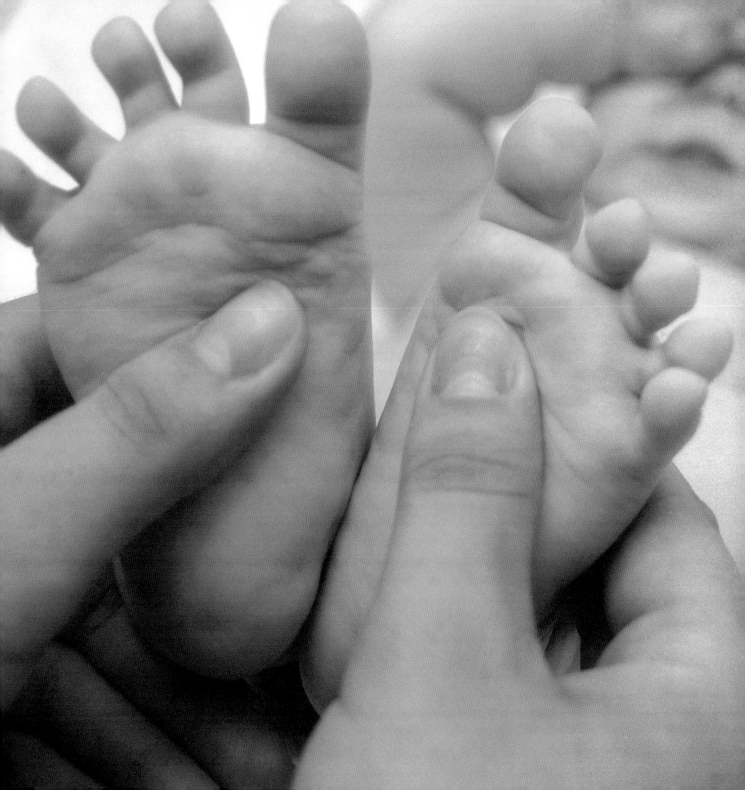

TADASANA

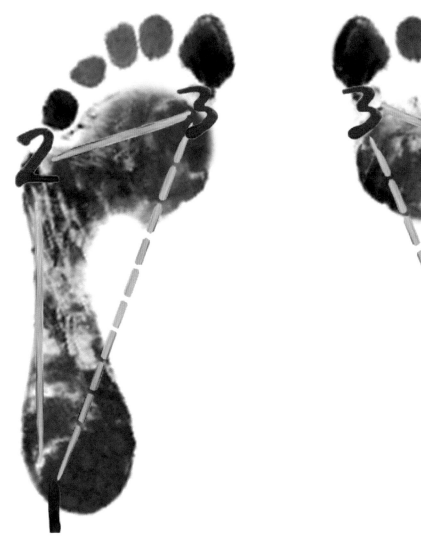
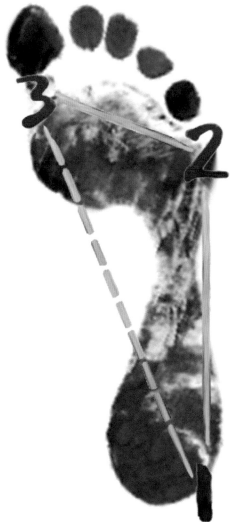

As you settle into standing, imagine looking up at the soles of your feet from the floor's point of view.

Envisage your exhalation travelling from the base of your brain down the spine and through the centre of your legs and out through the soles of your feet.

As you watch the breath leave, particularly allow:
- the heels (1) to drop into the floor.

- Following the line up the outside of the foot, release the base of the little toe (2) into the floor.

- Then also drop the base of the big toe (3) into the floor. You'll have given both feet an effective tripod base, supported by a natural arch.

Tip: Open your hands and fingers in the same way whilst you are trying to open your feet and toes. Doing the same movement with the hands makes copying it with the feet easier somehow.

TADASANA

When standing, imagine your feet growing bigger and bigger with every exhalation.
They become larger, softer and spongier as they settle into the floor.

This secure, heavy base allows the muscles surrounding the spine to release
and soften and you may experience a lengthening of your spine.

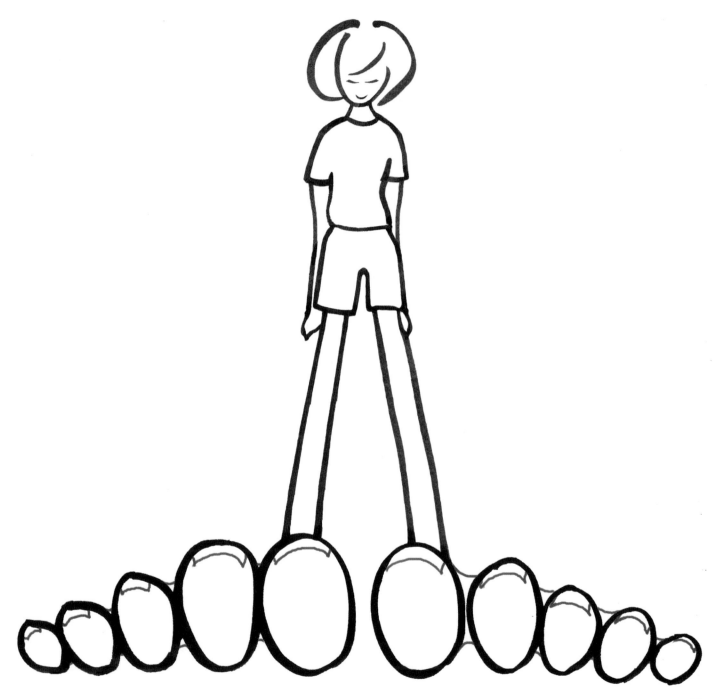

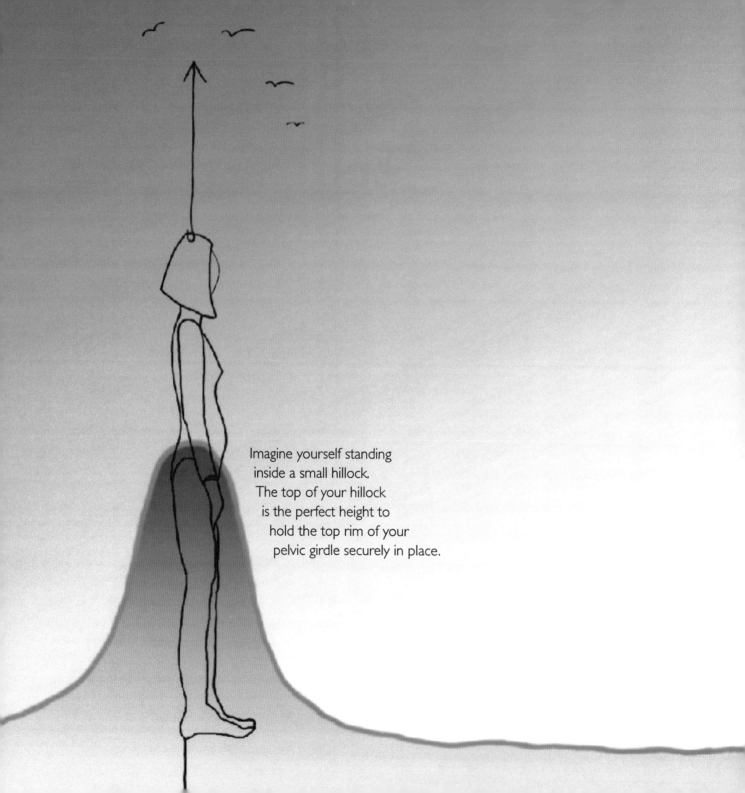

Imagine yourself standing
inside a small hillock.
The top of your hillock
is the perfect height to
hold the top rim of your
pelvic girdle securely in place.

STANDING / HILLOCK

TADASANA

As you breathe, see if you can pinpoint the exact moment that marks the end of an exhalation, when the strong feeling of groundedness is at its peak.

Look for an answering freedom in the spine.
The muscles around the spine gradually soften, allowing the individual vertebrae to move more independently.

Sometimes the downward sensation at the end of an exhalation sends an opening, rippling response upwards through the spine ... remember the bounce?

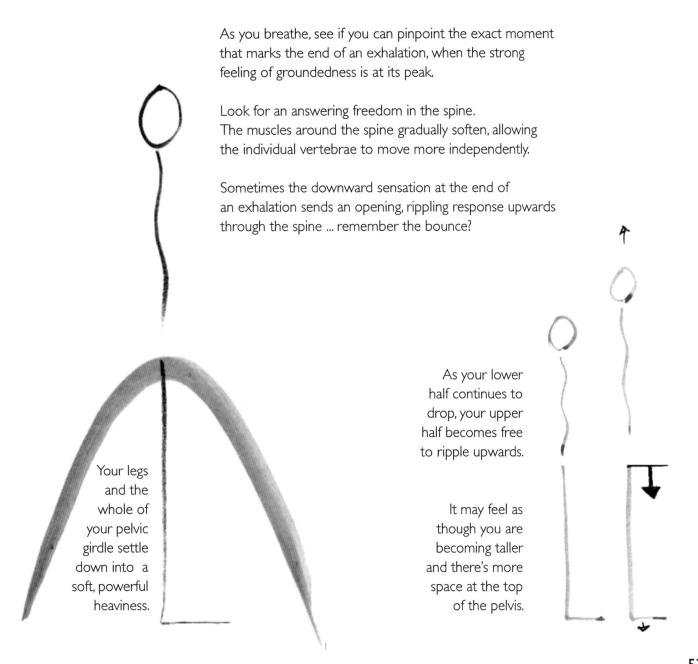

Your legs and the whole of your pelvic girdle settle down into a soft, powerful heaviness.

As your lower half continues to drop, your upper half becomes free to ripple upwards.

It may feel as though you are becoming taller and there's more space at the top of the pelvis.

TADASANA

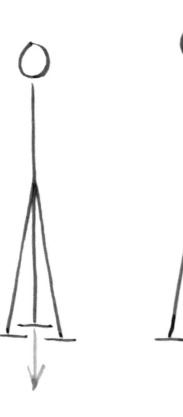

The more clearly you are able to visualise your tail, the firmer your whole base becomes.

When your tail feels well established, the whole upper body is now supported. It becomes free to open upwards - feeling softer and lighter.

When standing, visualise your exhalation travelling down the centre of your spine, through the tail bone and continuing downwards in the same direction - becoming a tail..

Watch your tail drop deeper and deeper beneath the floor, as it also grows, getting heavier and heavier...

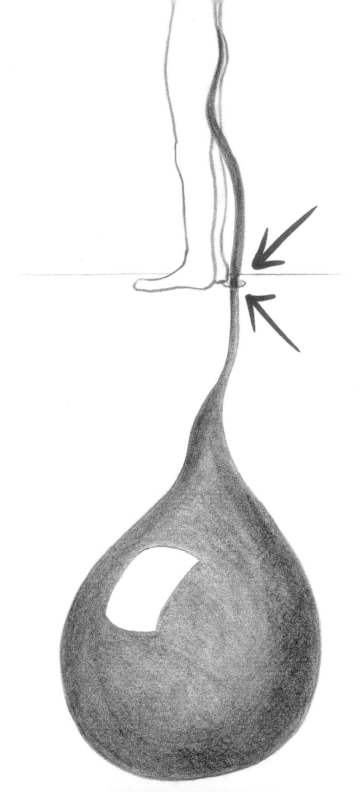

See if you can find the point on the ground where your 'tail' feels like it's dropping through the floor.

Keep imagining your tail growing bigger and heavier and dropping down deeper into the ground directly beneath you each time you breathe out.

The effect should be a base that feels heavy and solid but without tension.

RELAX

+ LET

YOUR

BONES

FIND

THEIR

OWN

WAY

HOME

TADASANA

A COUPLE OF IDEAS TO
HELP LENGTHEN THE NECK
WHEN STANDING

in the top centre of your head is a
hook attached to a pulley above.

the effect of the pulley pulling upwards while
allowing the shoulders to drop downwards
lengthens the space between the bottom
of the ears and the tops of the shoulders.

TADASANA

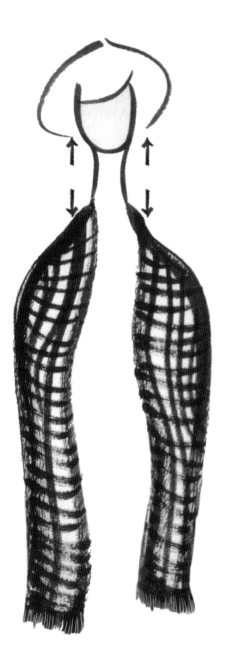

When standing (or sitting cross-legged), we want to release tension from our neck and shoulders.

Give yourself a heavy cape - maybe made of chain-mail, with particularly heavy weights at the bottom. Just let your shoulders release with gravity under the weight of the cape.

In time you'll find more space has been created between the bottom of the ears and the top of the shoulders.

Aaaaahhhhhhhhh

QUIETEN THE MIND
TO HELP YOU FEEL MORE CLEARLY

TADASANA

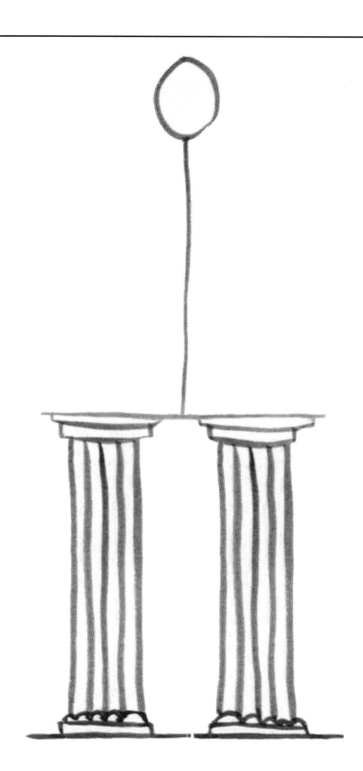

Another visualisation to help gravitate your lower half without tension ~

As you follow an exhalation travelling down the spine, out through the feet into the ground, watch your legs transform into two heavy pillars.

As you work with your attention to keep the visualisation solid, notice the stability having two pillars next to each other gives you.

weight can facilitate lightness

FORWARD BEND / LENGTHENING DOWN

UTTANASANA

1 Stand, breathing and grounding yourself from the top of your pelvis downwards.
Allow the upper body to soften and watch for the exact moment at the very end of an exhalation.

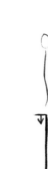

2 Let your spine 'catch' the rebound - feel it rippling up the spine like a snake. As the two halves of your body move away from each other, you may feel space opening up at the base of the spine - just above and around the sacrum.

3 At the end of an exhalation when your base is feeling well grounded, let your arms open upwards as lightly as you can, keeping your shoulders soft. Try not to let any tension into the upper body and do not disturb your roots.

4 Hinge slowly and gently down over a quiet pelvis.

Allow your top and bottom halves to keep on separating further.

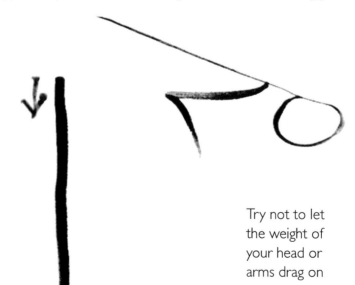

Try not to let the weight of your head or arms drag on your spine.

Keep breathing down evenly through the heels and all the toes.

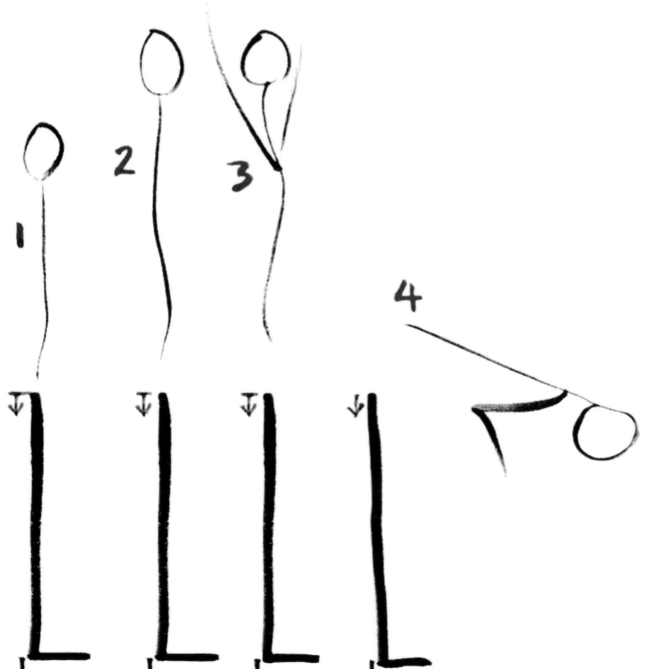

UTTANASANA

As you lengthen forward into
a forward bend, visualise your
pelvic girdle as a fan.
This fan has the potential to
open enormously - being pulled
in two directions; the weight of
the head vs the tail and heels
creating space all around the
sacrum and the lower spine.

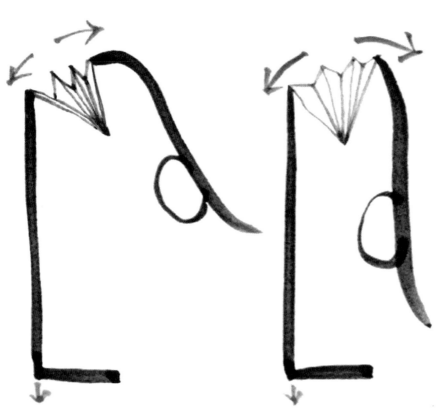

Keep your awareness
in your spine as you
'are breathed,' and see
if you can feel the
individual vertebrae
of your spine moving
away from each other.

As you
continue to lengthen forward,
the opening of the fan opens the
space around the sacrum. Feel the whole
lower back really begin to open
and soften.

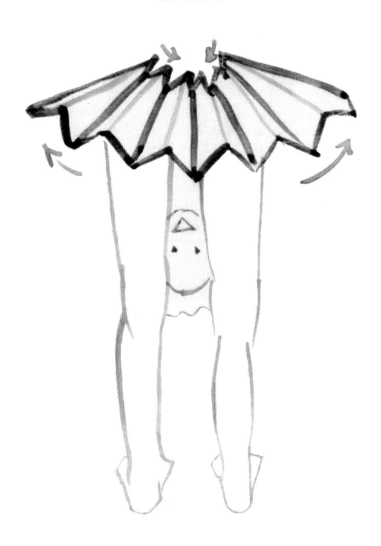

WATCH THE
TENSION MELT
AT THE END
OF AN EXHALATION

UTTANASANA

Behind your knees is a handily placed sunlamp. Obviously you'd like the backs of your knees to have a nice even tan - with no unsightly little white lines!

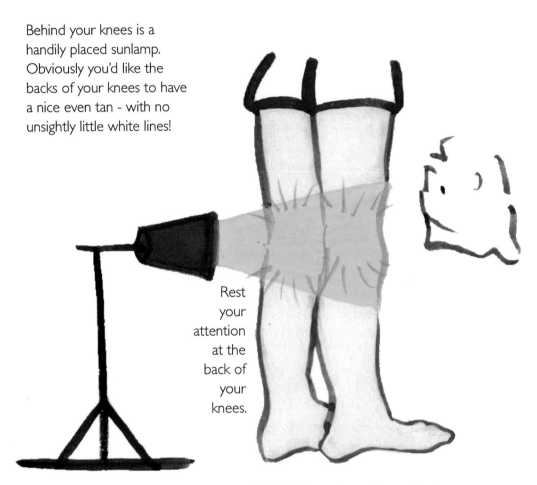

Rest your attention at the back of your knees.

Exhale down through your heels as you enjoy watching the backs of your knees softening in the warmth, keeping your kneecaps relaxed.

UTTANASANA

This is for people whose knees never fully open. If you have any tendency to hyper-extend the backs of your knees, don't do this - in fact always try to keep them slightly soft.

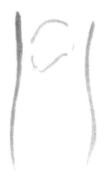

When you have relaxed the upper half of your body in forward bend and you're feeling calm and aligned, allow your kneecaps to engage and lift to open the backs of the knees more fully.

Try not to allow any other areas of the body to tense in sympathy.

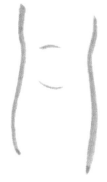

Carefully release the knee caps while keeping the backs of the knees soft and open.

Can you discern the direct relationship between the backs of the knees and the heels?

To keep your knees open without tensing the kneecaps, rest your attention at the back of the knees... just let it live there for a while.

You can try resting your attention on, or in, any part of the body which feels like it may benefit.

BE CALM
IN THE POSE

FORWARD BEND / INVISIBLE HELPER

UTTANASANA

As you may not always have an able and willing helper around, why not
have a go at creating your own?

Helpers are always just the right shape and size, are infinitely
patient and just as versatile as you want them to be:

in forward bend, the ideal helper is much
bigger than you and leans his weight
down onto your pelvic rim, while
also holding your heels down
nice and firmly.

Relax and
let go.

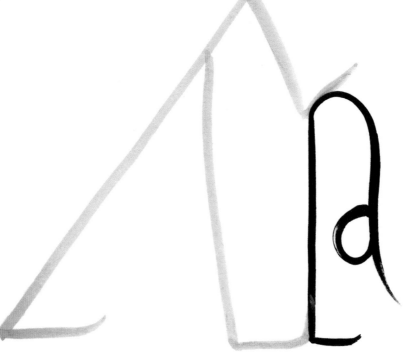

UTTANASANA

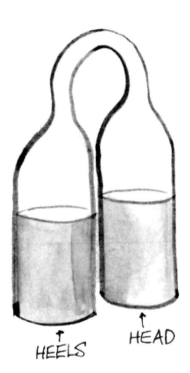

HEELS

HEAD

When you're in forward bend, it can feel like you have nearly as much weight in the head as the heels

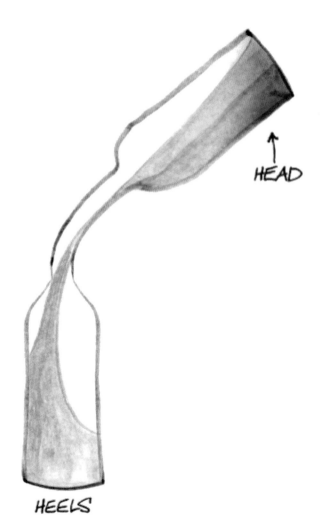

HEAD

HEELS

As you come up, it's as if all the weight you were holding in your upper body gets *poured into your base*

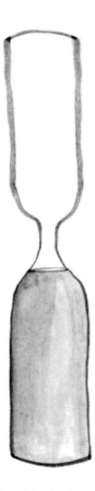

Standing again with all of your weight now
settled back in your lower half, the upper
body feels completely light and empty.

Aaaaaaaaaahhhhh

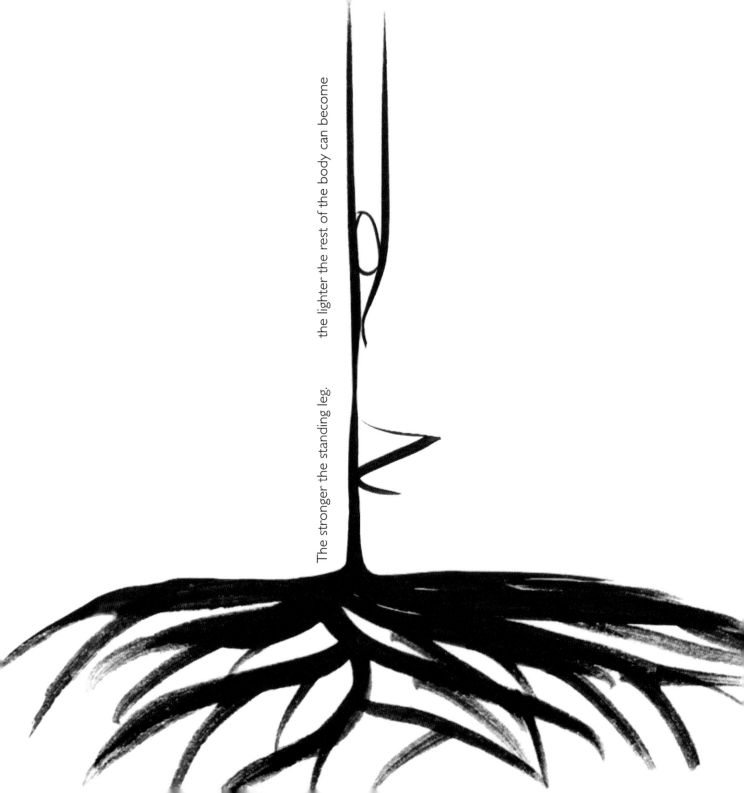

The stronger the standing leg, the lighter the rest of the body can become

TREE / ROOTS

VRIKASANA

Go into tree slowly.

When you're there, carefully watch an
exhalation as it travels down the very
centre of your spine and the standing leg.
As the breath enters the ground through
your massive standing foot, feel powerful
roots grow out through the sole of your
foot in all directions.

The leg feels increasingly like a rooted tree
trunk - stable yet passive.

The roots grow deeper, wider and stronger
with each exhalation.

TRIANGLE / G-CLAMP

TRIKONASANA

Triangle has incredible potential to twist the spine in some very hard-to-reach places...

... yet it can easily become just another hamstring stretch if you allow your top hip to stick out.

As you go down into the pose, visualise a G-clamp on your back hip, holding it exactly in place.

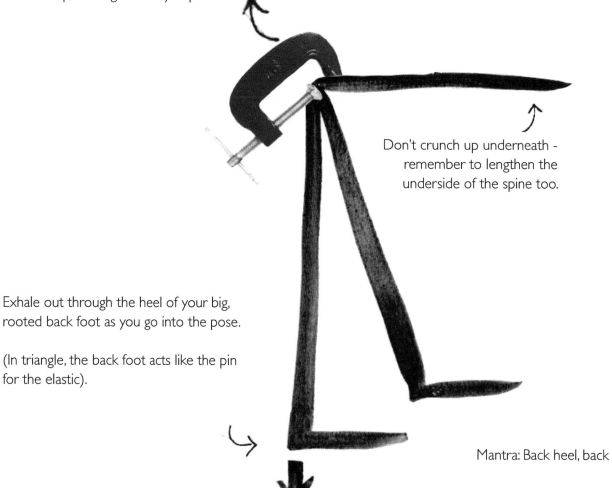

Don't crunch up underneath - remember to lengthen the underside of the spine too.

Exhale out through the heel of your big, rooted back foot as you go into the pose.

(In triangle, the back foot acts like the pin for the elastic).

Mantra: Back heel, back

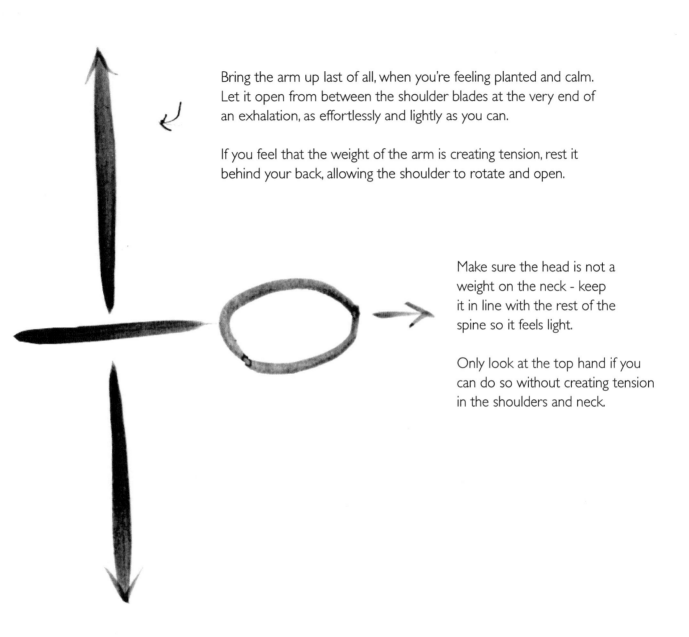

Bring the arm up last of all, when you're feeling planted and calm. Let it open from between the shoulder blades at the very end of an exhalation, as effortlessly and lightly as you can.

If you feel that the weight of the arm is creating tension, rest it behind your back, allowing the shoulder to rotate and open.

Make sure the head is not a weight on the neck - keep it in line with the rest of the spine so it feels light.

Only look at the top hand if you can do so without creating tension in the shoulders and neck.

heel, back heel, back heel, back heel, back heel, back heel, back heel, back heel...

TRIANGLE / DOUBLE GLAZING

TRIKONASANA

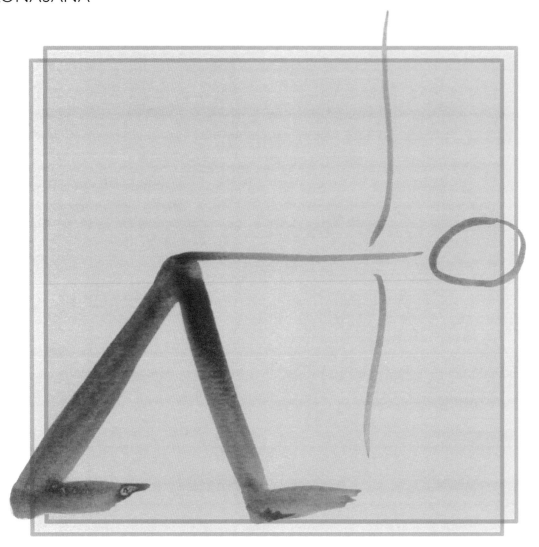

A common difficulty in triangle is keeping the spine in line with the
legs, there's a natural tendency to reach forwards as we go down.
So try imagining yourself held between two large sheets
of glass - it's like being supported inside giant double glazing.

IT'S JUST
ANOTHER
POSITION
TO BE
BREATHED IN

DOG / PULLEY

ADHO MUKHA SVANASANA

Dog pose gives your spine the chance to be as long as it can be.
But the muscles around the spine have to soften for this to be pleasurable.

Check your throat and chest and shoulders feel relaxed before you start...

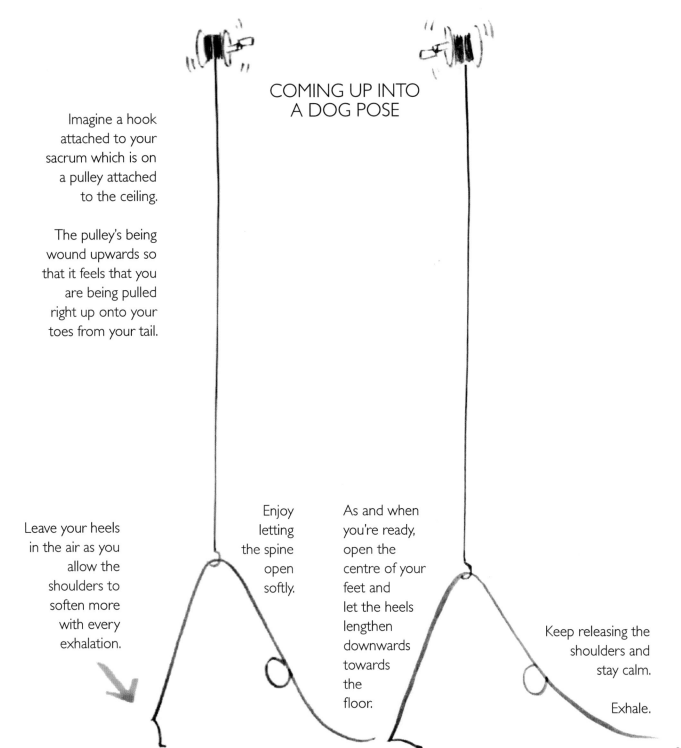

COMING UP INTO A DOG POSE

Imagine a hook attached to your sacrum which is on a pulley attached to the ceiling.

The pulley's being wound upwards so that it feels that you are being pulled right up onto your toes from your tail.

Leave your heels in the air as you allow the shoulders to soften more with every exhalation.

Enjoy letting the spine open softly.

As and when you're ready, open the centre of your feet and let the heels lengthen downwards towards the floor.

Keep releasing the shoulders and stay calm.

Exhale.

DOG / BOXING GLOVE

ADHO MUKHA SVANASANA

Once your tail bone has been lifted upwards and you come to settle
into dog pose, try imagining a boxing glove gently nestling into your
lower abdomen, supporting you from underneath.

Watch for the moment at the very end of the exhalation, when the
lungs are empty and the diaphragm is pulled up and widens,
engaging the deep abdominal muscles.

Now you're free to allow your shoulders to soften and maybe for your
feet to open a bit so the heels can drop towards the floor.
Notice the relationship between the heels and the backs of the knees.

Soften your shoulders, neck and throat as you exhale.

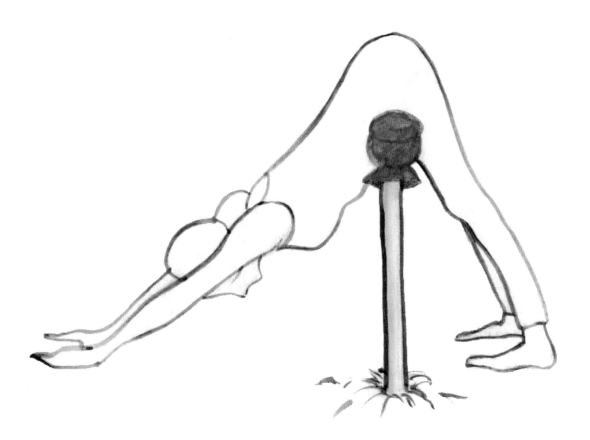

ADHO MUKHA SVANASANA

Once you're settled into the dog pose and feel supported from underneath,
you may choose to see how softly and calmly you can stay there.

If you want to work a bit more in the pose, imagine that your thigh bones are
growing and lengthening along their current axis... upwards and upwards.

Lengthening seems to happen most easily at the end of an exhalation.

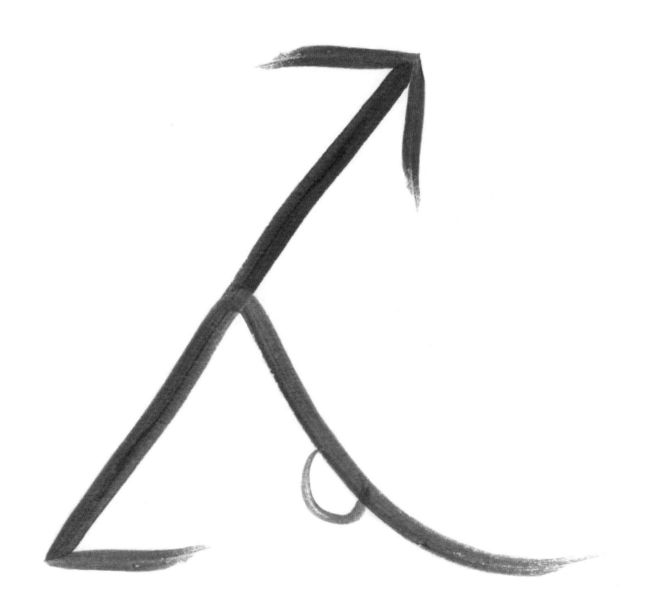

COBRA / BABY

BHUJANGASANA

Yoga at its best can feel like regaining the ease and openness
we had in our bodies when we were babies.

Cobra can be a particularly good example of this. When you watch a
baby the usual barriers to adult back-bending simply don't occur:
- babies allow their legs to be naturally heavy with the muscles relaxed.
- the base of a baby's throat and the chest itself are completely soft
and ready to open
- notice also how the baby's neck is simply the continuation of the
spine; the head is not thrown back so the throat isn't stretched.

When practising cobra, spend time allowing your deep abdominal
muscles to be engaged with the exhalation. We all need to lengthen
our tailbones and engage our deep core in any kind of backbend to
protect the lower vertebrae from getting squashed and damaged.

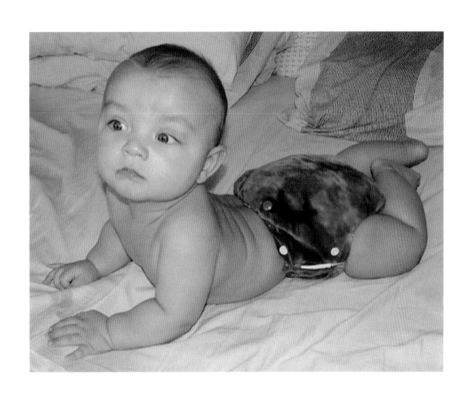

URDHVA DHANURASANA

Take your time preparing for a back-bend.

The base of the throat, the chest including the heart, the solar plexus and the whole of the stomach and pelvis should be 'emptied' of tension first. Conjure up some 'little helpers' to help ...

They carry away the heavy weight of anxiety and attach it to a heavy weight directly under the feet - particularly the heels.

As you continue to empty your upper body and visualise your feet dropping into the ground, your pelvis may lift off the floor - *as if from under your heels.* Keep checking that you're not tensing the shoulders as you do this and keep following your diaphragm as it lifts and widens strongly with the exhalation.

NOTE: For many people this preparation is in itself a sufficient back-bend - do not continue to full backbend unless you know what you're doing!

Experienced practitioners find that the deep abdomen
becomes engaged by the end of the exhalation causing the
navel to move back in towards the front of the spine and
the sacrum to move forwards.
Great - but don't let the shoulders, chest stomach or pelvis
become tight as a result!

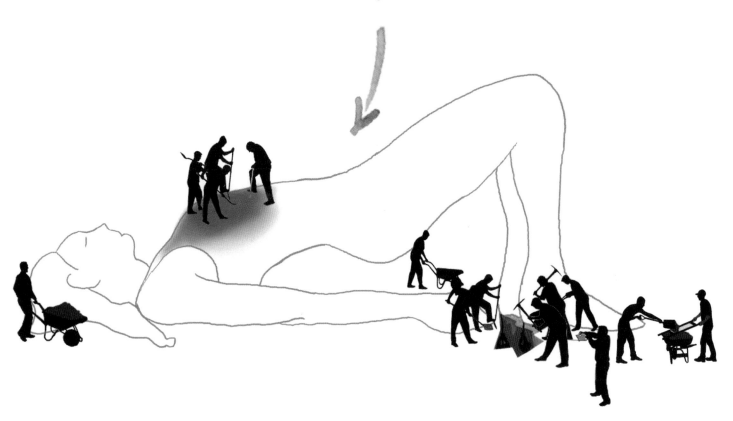

BACKBEND / FEET MEN

URDHVA DHANURASANA

Don't be in a hurry to go up.

Take your time resting deeply on the floor, breathing all
tension out of the neck, throat, shoulders and chest.
Spend as long as you like emptying the pelvis too.

All this energy is directed to the area where your feet
meet the floor - deepen that connection as you exhale...

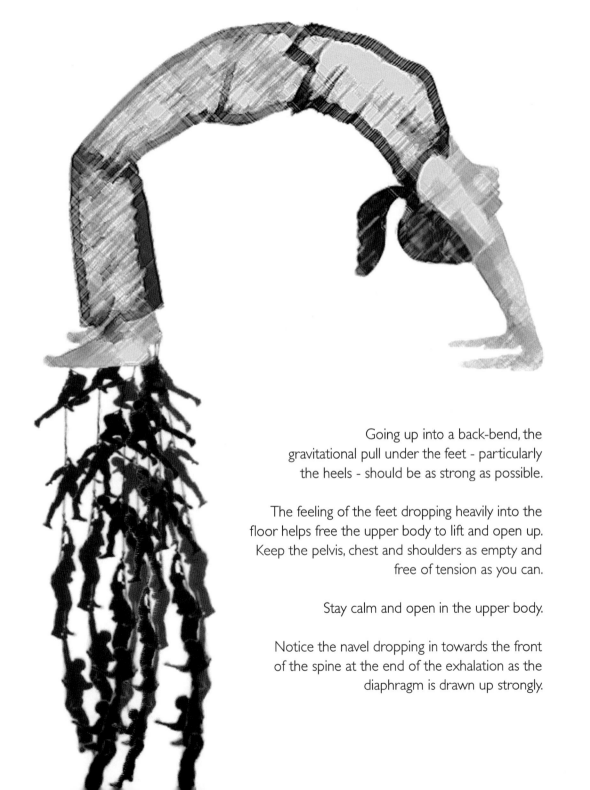

Going up into a back-bend, the gravitational pull under the feet - particularly the heels - should be as strong as possible.

The feeling of the feet dropping heavily into the floor helps free the upper body to lift and open up. Keep the pelvis, chest and shoulders as empty and free of tension as you can.

Stay calm and open in the upper body.

Notice the navel dropping in towards the front of the spine at the end of the exhalation as the diaphragm is drawn up strongly.

CHILD'S POSE / INVISIBLE SITTER

SUPTA VAJRASANA

Child's pose can be treated as an active posture.
Usually though, we use it as a resting position, releasing the spine and shoulders completely.

It's really pleasant and also helpful to have someone putting
weight on the top of your pelvis, keeping your hips from rising up.

If you don't have anyone handy, just imagine a 'heavy helper' instead.

Keep releasing the shoulder blades as you breathe out.

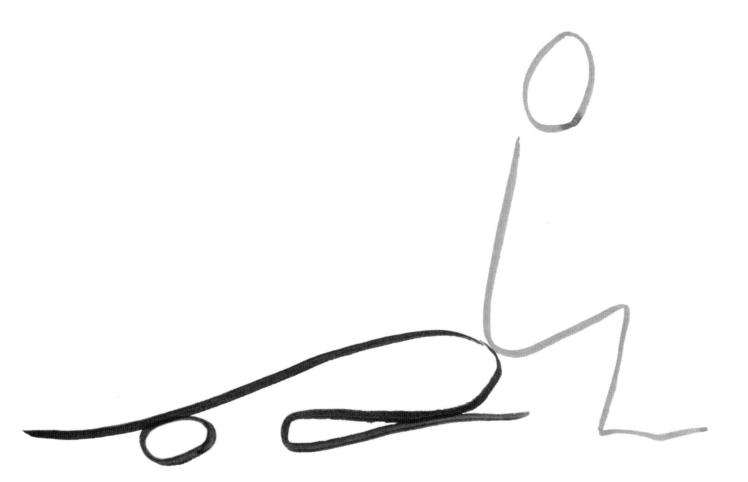

SARVANGASANA

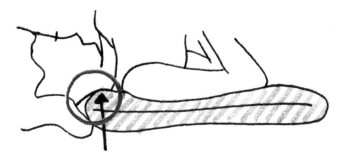

Rest the base of your brain (cerebellum) on the edge of a thick
blanket, so that your arms fit comfortably on the same blanket
and your head rests on a mat.

Keep rotating the upper arms outwards -
opening the heart area.
Then wait, becoming calmer as you breathe
and relax the neck and shoulders.

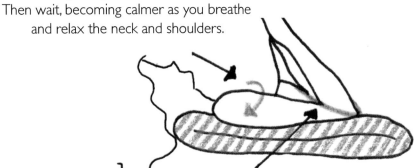

Optional; in order to keep the elbows
close together comfortably, tie with a strap.

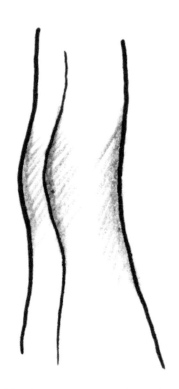

The kneecaps stay released.
Don't allow tension in the
legs or pelvis as you
continue to release the neck
and shoulders into the floor.

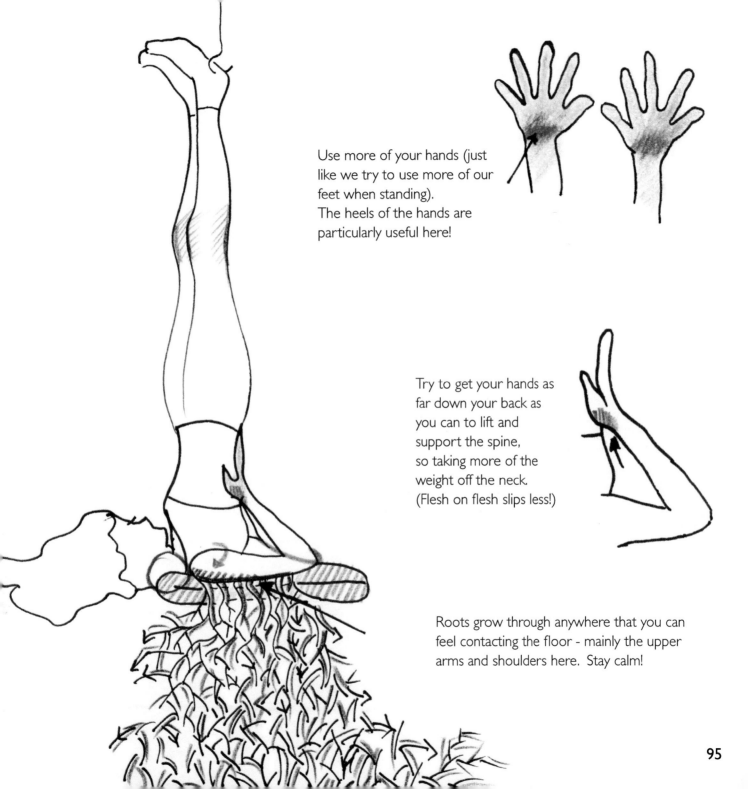

Use more of your hands (just like we try to use more of our feet when standing).
The heels of the hands are particularly useful here!

Try to get your hands as far down your back as you can to lift and support the spine, so taking more of the weight off the neck. (Flesh on flesh slips less!)

Roots grow through anywhere that you can feel contacting the floor - mainly the upper arms and shoulders here. Stay calm!

95

UPAVISTHA KONASANA

Spend some time sitting up straight with your legs wide open and dropping into the floor before you start to lean forward. Go through the whole body, checking for and releasing tension.

Focus your attention away from where you're facing to the other leg - and let that back leg 'go' so that it feels like it's detaching itself from you at the groin. Release that back leg enough and it may even feel like it starts to move away from you - rather like a log floating off downstream.

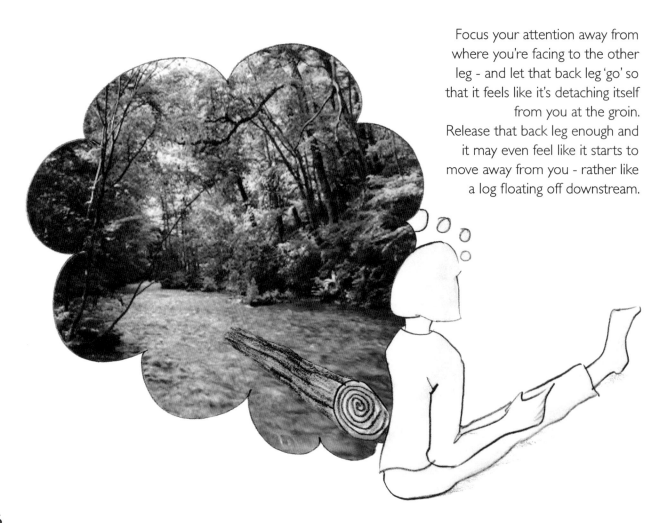

When the pelvis is released equally on both sides, turn to the side you're going
to bend over and focus your attention entirely on the other leg.

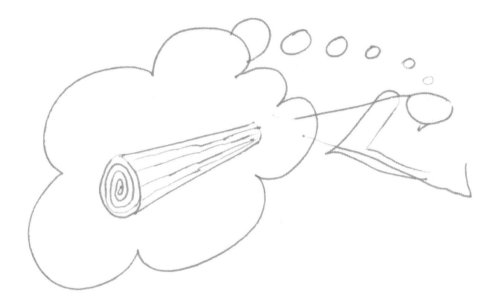

Visualise your back leg having detached itself from your pelvis,
now floating like a log downstream, away from you.

A slightly odd side-effect of this visualisation is that it becomes easier
to release the blockage that was preventing you from softening over
the front leg as you gently hinge downwards.

Don't try to force yourself down over the legs;
just exhale and look for any extra range of movement you're
'given' at the end of the exhalation.

FEAR OF TENSION
IN THE MUSCLES...

CAUSES TENSION
IN THE MUSCLES.

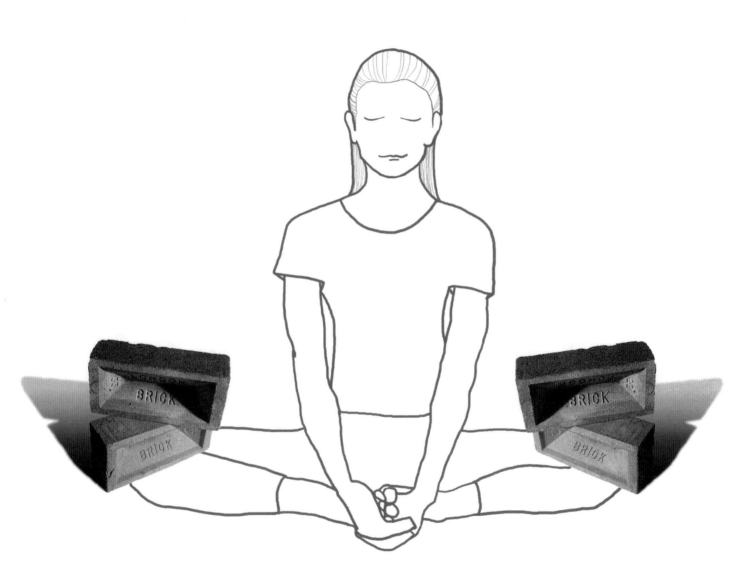

SIRSASANA

The same 'hillock' visualisation used in standing can
also be helpful when sitting in any crossed-leg position.
We want everything from the top of the pelvis
downwards to drop into the floor, releasing the upper
body so it can soften and lengthen, opening upwards.

Look for the the exact moment that marks the very
end of any exhalation. At that moment allow the hips
and legs to really drop, softening heavily into the floor.
Immediately after that dropping, look for a wave-like
response in the spine that ripples upwards towards
the sky. The head lifts from the very centre of the top
of your head, lengthening the neck.

The passive spine responds to these two opposing forces
by opening gently - particularly around the lower vertebrae.

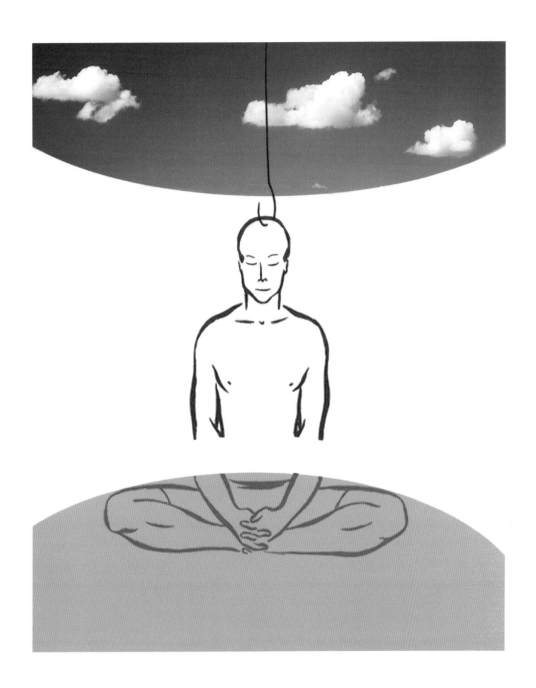

SITTING / HANGING TAIL

e.g. ARDHA PADMASANA (half lotus)

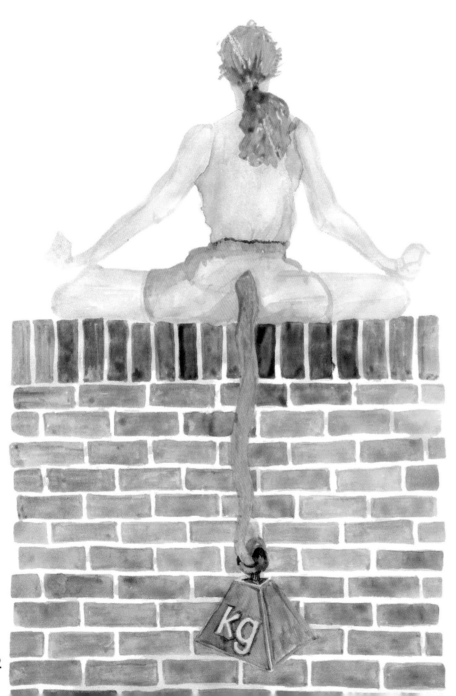

When sitting in any crossed leg position, once your legs begin to feel heavy and your groin muscles begin to release, it can be helpful to imagine that you are sitting on a wall...

you have a tail hanging down over the wall with a heavy weight attached to it.

Allow all the muscles in the pelvis and thighs to melt with the exhalation as your tail keeps dropping, becoming heavier with each breath.

SAVOUR
THE
SILENCE
OF
THE
POSE

CORPSE POSE / MELTING BUTTER

SAVASANA

This pose could have come at the beginning or the end as I always finish a
practice with a version of corpse pose and often start with it too.
There are loads of great visuals for relaxation, but I do like the simplicity of melting.

Having internally 'patrolled' the body, releasing tension bit by bit, have the idea of
simply allowing your body to melt as a whole into the floor.
As you continue to let go ...deeper and deeper... you'll feel like your body is
spreading into the ground, your backprint literally taking more and more space.

Enjoy watching all your muscle tension melt into gravity with an easy breath.

Bliss.

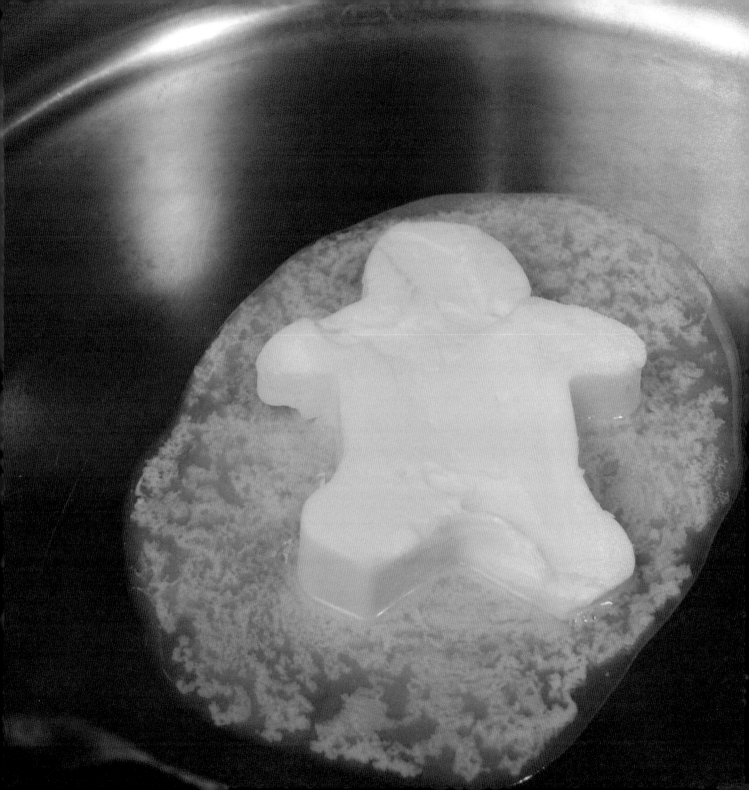

TEACHERS WHO MADE A DIFFERENCE

VANDA SCARAVELLI

I was lucky enough to meet Vanda in 1991. I won't begin to try to explain her work here, but if you haven't already, do read her book "Awakening the Spine". She showed us that yoga really could and should be pleasurable. To work with the body, never against it. That being soft doesn't mean being lazy. To listen more. That our spines really can dance to the breath if we pay attention and so much more.

JOHN STIRK

John has been my primary teacher since 1987. It's through him I met both Vanda Scaravelli and Sandra Sabatini and I often hear his voice in my head when I practise. I owe him a great deal. Many of his ideas appear in one shape or another throughout this book - though I have to stress that I take responsibility for exactly what is said here and how!
John Stirk is a gifted teacher. He is known for his knowledge of anatomy as he is also a respected osteopath, which tends to make his teaching detailed and anatomically specific. His teaching goes deeper than most and changes constantly, sometimes working with utter softness and at other times really challenging inner strength. Long may this fascinating journey continue!
He has published two books: 'Soft Exercise: The Complete Book of Stretching' and 'Structural Fitness'.

SANDRA SABATINI

Sandra is an inspirational teacher. She worked closely with Vanda for 17 years and has gone on to share and develop Vanda's ideas in a unique way. I have mostly worked with Sandra over longer periods - typically workshops, where she gently brings her students to stillness and clarity. With Sandra, the breath and the postures are completely inseparable. Her first book is called 'Breath, the Essence of Yoga' and her latest (co-authored) book is entitled: Autumn, Winter, Spring, Summer; Yoga Through The Seasons.

SU SAREEN

Su Sareen began learning yoga with Iyengar trained teachers in 1978, but it wasn't until after the natural birth of her first child, when the awesome power of yoga became apparent, that yoga became more central to her life. When she realised the beauty, simplicity and effectiveness of Vanda Scaravelli's insights, she became determined to share these ideas. She started to teach yoga in 1991 and has taught continuously (part-time), ever since.

Meanwhile, Su also worked as an advertising art director – then creative director, and won many top international creative awards. She has also directed TV commercials and pop promo's and worked as a documentary director at the BBC. Now running her own digital creative company, she continues to teach yoga.

Su has been trained to summarise ideas clearly and simply and to communicate them in easy-to-understand, compelling and visually memorable ways. This book is the outcome of this unusual combination of years of experience communicating ideas visually with 30 years of yoga practice.

Yoga is a journey - we never reach an ending.
This book represents where Su happens to be on that journey now.

ISBN: 144043848X
EAN: 9781440438486

Made in the USA
Charleston, SC
07 November 2010